Adventures in Neurology

An 11-Year-Old's Perspective

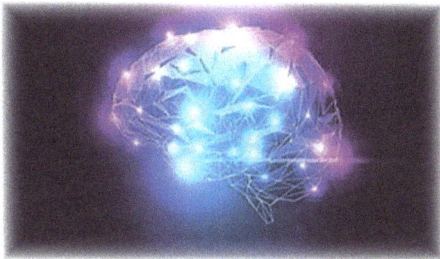

Braydon Joshua Dominique

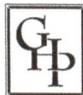

Grosvenor House
Publishing Limited

This book is published by
Grosvenor House Publishing Ltd
Link House
140 The Broadway, Tolworth, Surrey, KT6 7HT.
www.grosvenorhousepublishing.co.uk

A CIP record for this book
is available from the British Library

Paperback ISBN 978-1-83615-063-3
Hardback ISBN 978-1-83615-064-0

Disclaimer:

This book is written by a 12-year-old author and is intended for informational
and educational purposes only. The content provided in this book is based on
research from various sources, as well as the author's personal understanding
and interpretation of Alzheimer's, Parkinson's, and Huntington's diseases.
While every effort has been made to present accurate and up-to-date
information, the author is not a medical professional.

Readers are strongly encouraged to consult qualified healthcare
professionals for any medical concerns, diagnoses, or treatment options
related to these conditions. This book should not be used as a
substitute for professional medical advice, diagnosis, or treatment.
The author and publisher are not responsible for any actions taken
based on the information provided in this book.

*I dedicate this book to all
the young people interested
in science out there, come
and join the field of neurology*

Table of Contents

Summary

Introduction: In this book lies a journey into the intricate depths of neurological disorders—Parkinson's, Alzheimer's, and Huntington's diseases. Created for the discerning minds of potential scientists, researchers, and medical practitioners, this book serves as a fountain of knowledge.

Section 1: Parkinson's Disease Delving into the realm of Parkinson's disease, I first introduce its fundamental nature—a degenerative disorder of the central nervous system characterised by motor impairments, tremors, and rigidity.

Section 2: Alzheimer's Disease The narrative then unfolds to unveil the enigma of Alzheimer's disease—a progressive neurodegenerative disorder marked by cognitive decline, memory loss, and behavioural changes. Throughout this section, I introduce the current medicines, and from there, I explain.

Section 3: Huntington's Disease As the journey progresses, the spotlight turns towards Huntington's disease—a genetic condition characterised by involuntary movements, cognitive impairment, and emotional disturbances. Here, you are immersed in the deep world of genetics, and I give a detailed explanation of what causes the diseases and the components that characterise them.

Conclusion: As the journey draws to a close, readers emerge enlightened and armed with a deeper understanding of Parkinson's, Alzheimer's, and Huntington's diseases. This book is constructed from scratch with passion and knowledge; I hope it serves as a guiding light for future endeavours in scientific inquiry and medical innovation, propelling us ever closer to unravelling the mysteries of the human mind.

Advanced Neuroprotection in Parkinson's

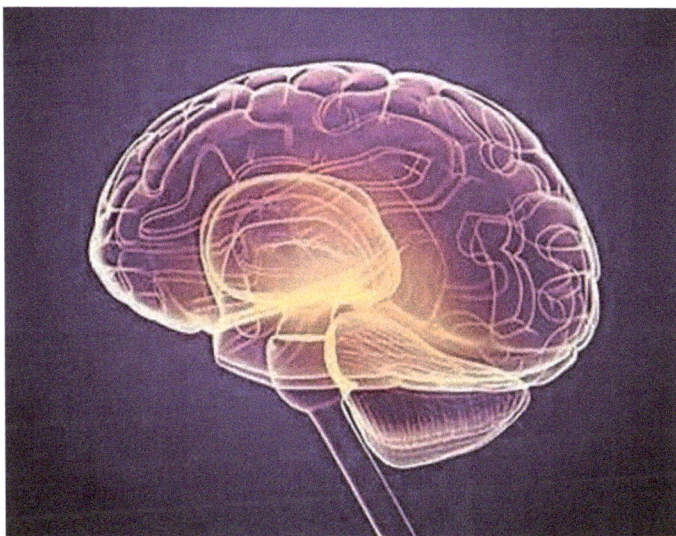

History of Parkinson's

This earliest traces of the disease was as early as 1000 BC in India, some medical accounts were written about it classified under an unknown name and was treated with the ancient Indian remedies of Aruyveda. It was described as short tremors and difficulty to move highlighting the diseases well known symptom traits. Doing some research on the Aruyveda techniques to avoid Kampavata (name given to Parkinsons in Aruyveda) the remedies might not have been as absurd as we may have thought. The word 'Kampa' means tremors and the word 'Vata' which is the word associated with the nervous system in Aruyveda. It is believe ed to be caused by aggravating the Vata dosha with an array of things such as an unhealthy lifestyle, excess caffeine intake and a lot of stress. There are few herbal remedies, the one which stood out the most to me was **Kapikachhu** which has naturally occurring levodopa to help restore dopamine in the brain which is a key factor in Parkinsons I will talk about later on.

Later on the English surgeon James Parkinsons wrote a ground breaking essay titled 'An Essay on the Shaking Palsy' in 1817 where he highlighted six cases of people that displayed similar symptoms of tremor and linked them under one disease. He was the first person to provide a foundation of the research of the disease.

Jean-Martin-Charcot often referred to as the father of modern neurology named the disease as Parkinson's disease relating to James Parkinsons's work on the disease and helped differentiate it from other diseases with similar tremors as to those described commonly in Parkinson's.

In the early 20th century more research was done into the brain anatomy, this when the basal ganglia was discovered, this is a group of nuclei which affects the motor control of the brain, they discovered that in this part of the brain and a part called the substania nigra cells producing an important neurotransmitter called dopamine were dying due to factors I will explain later on.

A lot of research and work has been put into trying to cure the disease, as I have personal experience knowing someone with the disease I see the changes that must be made to their lifestyle, the physical and mental effect it has on them and their family. Parkinson's patients often find talking about the disease quite challenging as it is a very sensitive topic, however with my own research I have found out about the disease and the current medicines being used to treat it.

What is Parkinson's Disease and what Causes It?

Parkinson's Disease is a neurodegenerative disease that normally affects people over 50. Parkinson's Disease is caused by the loss of dopaminergic neurons produced in the substantia nigra and the ventral tegmental area, which are both situated near the rear middle part of the brain. These neurons produce a substance called dopamine, also known as the 'reward chemical'. Dopamine is classified as a neurotransmitter that allows nerve cells to communicate (like a messenger); it coordinates and controls movements in the body. When dopamine is lost in the body, it can lead to various neurological diseases, one of the most dangerous of which is Parkinson's.

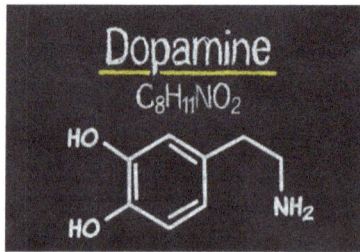

Dopamine
$C_8H_{11}NO_2$

What Causes Dopamine Loss?

Dopamine loss is caused by the loss or depletion of dopaminergic neurons, which are destroyed through aging, oxidative stress, or genetics. However, in Parkinson's, abnormal protein clumps called Lewy bodies disrupt the cells' functions, which eventually leads to cell death. Lewy bodies are created by a protein called alpha-synuclein, which is normally found in neurons in the brain. When alpha-synuclein undergoes a process called misfolding, it forms Lewy bodies. How Lewy bodies are created is not fully understood. but this process likely includes many factors, such as genetics, stress, and health conditions. These lumps of protein are normally present in the cytoplasm (the part of the cell where chemical reactions occur). They can be viewed through a microscope and appear as irregular circular shapes.

SUBSTANTIA NIGRA

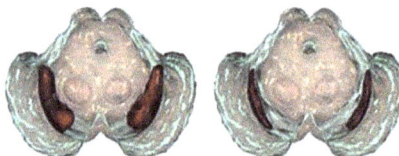

Normal   Parkinson's disease

What are the Symptoms of Dopamine Loss?

Many factors contribute to dopamine loss, and I explain them all in detail below.

Genetics

Genetics plays a huge role in dopamine loss. However, the main aspect that most people do not understand is that you are not guaranteed to never develop Parkinson's just because your father or mother did not have it. Directly inheriting Parkinson's is possible, but this is very rarely the reason for developing Parkinson's. Rather. it develops through other symptoms of dopamine loss. For example, if your uncle has gastrointestinal problems, then you have a chance of developing Parkinson's. This is because you could inherit the same gastrointestinal problems. which is a symptom of dopamine loss, and if this symptom gradually becomes worse alongside other symptoms, such as stress and lack of sleep, the final result could be dopamine loss. This can be described as genetic interlinking.

Restless Leg Syndrome

Restless leg syndrome (RLS) occurs when you have the strong urge to move your legs when resting, and you may also feel itching, pulling, crawling, and throbbing in your legs. It normally occurs in the evening when resting. These are the main symptoms of this syndrome, as it is not caused by any other medical conditions. Another similar symptom that causes RLS and Parkinson's is stress. RLS can also be inherited genetically and often leads to dopamine loss indirectly, similar to the example in the previous section.

Triggers

Caffeine → Coffee
Alcohol → For example, whiskey, wine, and brandy
Nicotine → Chemical produced from smoking
Stress → General stress

Gastrointestinal Problems

Some gastrointestinal problems cause your bowel movements to be less frequent, and when you do go to the toilet, it often causes pain. This could be because of the formation of Lewy bodies in the gut, which could travel up the vascular tube connecting the gut to the brain and then affect the brain.

Weak Peripheral Nervous System

The peripheral nervous system (PNS) is made up of your brain and spinal cord as well as the peripheral nerves, which connect the first two organs to the rest of the body. Patients with Parkinson's often have a weak PNS. The PNS helps the body send signals and react to the surroundings, but as Parkinson's disease has the exact opposite effect, the PNS in patients with Parkinson's is not very strong.

Other Symptoms

A few other symptoms are linked to dopamine loss, but they are not 'major players' like the ones listed above.

These include:

- Lack of motivation
- Fatigue

- Low concentration level and span (may be linked to attention-deficit/hyperactivity disorder, ADHD)
- Moodiness and anxiousness
- Not much pleasure from remembering or recalling previous enjoyable experiences (may link to schizophrenia)
- Depression and hopelessness (may be linked to schizophrenia)
- Low sex drive (may be linked with trouble sleeping)
- Trouble sleeping (may be linked with a low sex drive)
- Hand tremors
- Short-term memory
- Lack of problem-solving skills
- Trouble remembering daily routines
- Anxiety
- Lack of organisation skills
- Acting quickly

Current Cures and Remedies

Many medicines can help reduce the living difficulties of Parkinson's disease. These medicines mainly aim to make life easier rather than to cure the disease. The two main variants of dopamine that are used as replacements for dopamine loss are levodopa and dopamine agonists. I explain these two in detail below.

Levodopa

Levodopa is a variant of dopamine that acts like dopamine on the dopamine receptors and helps the body run smoothly for a period of time. Levodopa works by crossing the blood–brain barrier and then converting to dopamine and boosting the dopamine levels in the brain. Although it is an effective treatment, it does not in any way halt Parkinson's disease from progressing. Levodopa is normally preferred over dopamine agonists because it offers more relief and acts more quickly.

Dopamine Agonists

Even though dopamine agonists act more slowly than levodopa, they have a longer duration of action, despite their painful side effects, which levodopa also has. The four main dopamine agonists used for Parkinson's that I found in my research are:

- Pramipexole
- Ropinirole
- Rotigotine
- Apomorphine

Pramipexole

Like a mechanic, this dopamine agonist identifies what is wrong in the complex wiring system of neurons. It then identifies the areas in the system that are weaker and restores conductivity between specific neurons to help them serve their purpose better and return the body to normal with suitable healthy neurons.

Ropinirole

This dopamine agonist is similar to pramipexole, but in my opinion, it is more effective. This is because ropinirole rearranges all of the neurotransmitter receptors so that everything runs smoothly in the body.

Rotigotine

Rotigotine is administered through a patch that is placed on the body to help dopamine-producing neurons grow, making them more effective and helping them produce more dopamine. This helps make up for the dopamine that is lost when dopaminergic neurons are depleted.

Apomorphine

This dopamine agonist works a bit like pramipexole as well; it locates the specific 'faulty' receptors and sends a surge of neurotransmitter activity through them. This dopamine agonist is popular because it has the quickest effect.

My Favourite Dopamine Agonist

In my opinion, the dopamine agonist that works the best is rotigotine. All dopamine agonists are incredible discoveries that have helped advance Parkinson's treatment, but rotigotine stood out to me because it helps the neurons that are already producing dopamine to produce more dopamine, which could greatly help relieve Parkinson's symptoms. I think pramipexole would work well with rotigotine because of its ability to identify problems and help restore the conductivity of specific neurons. One medicine would help the already healthy neurons produce more, and the other would help restore the conditions of the weaker ones.

The Most Effective Remedy (In My Opinion)

I think levodopa administered with rotigotine and pramipexole would be a good combination that would tackle most areas of Parkinson's. It would not necessarily cure Parkinson's disease, but it could offer tremendous symptom relief.

Levodopa + rotigotine + pramipexole → Excellent remedy for symptom relief

Alzheimer's Disease

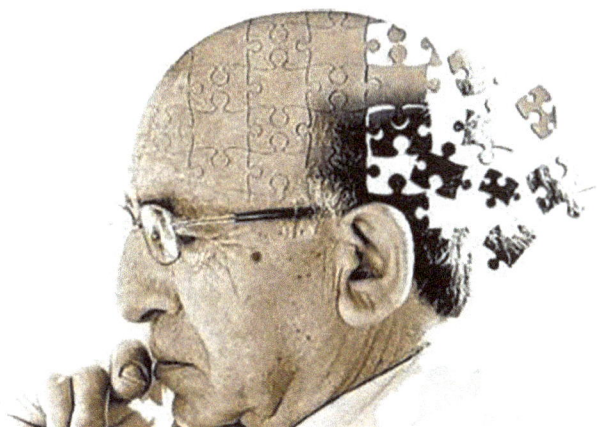

History of Alzheimers

Alzheimers was first discovered in 1901 in a patient called Auguste Deter. She was admitted into the Anstalt fur Irre und Epeliptische translated Asylum for Lunatics and Epileptics by her husband after he reported her experiencing memory loss, decline in various cognitive functions and disorientation. A physicatarian Alois Alzheimier was surprised at this case of a 51 year old displaying symptoms of dementia.

An example conservation between Alois and Auguste would have went like this:

What's your name?	'Auguste'
Family name?	'Auguste'
'What's your husbands name?' –	
she hesitates finally answers	'I believe … Auguste'
'Your husband?'	'Oh my husband'
How are old you	Fifty-one
Are you married	Oh I am so confused

After her death Alois asked for her brain to be extracted and when searching her brain he came across abnormal plaques and tangles that seemed to be made from some sort of protein. He presented this finding in an conference in 1906.

Alois apprentice Emil Kraepelin named this disease after Alois in it's 1910 publication.

In the early 1970's Alzheimers was a common name to describe common dementia in older adults. After some development the amyloid theory was proposed, this theory highlighted that beta amyloid plaques were one of the main reasons that Alzheimer's Disease was so deadly.

In 1990's more research was done on the genetic side of Alzheimer's as they identified which gene would have been mutated to produce the beta amyloid plaques.

In 2010 PET scans were improved in order to identify beta amyloid plaques and tau tangles in the brain.

Overall significant improvement has been made in Alzheimers disease and I will be highlighting the most popular treatments later on.

What is Alzheimer's Disease and what Causes It?

Alzheimer's disease is a neurodegenerative disease that, because of many factors, causes the brain to shrink and the brain cells to eventually die. The exact cause of Alzheimer's disease is not known, but it is said to involve many factors, such as genetics, oxidative stress, neuroinflammation, tau tangles, build-up of beta-amyloid plaques, and the excessive release of glutamate.

Acetylcholine

This is a neurotransmitter that helps with memory and learning, as it helps people recall previous experiences and remember normal routines by accessing them through connecting neurons responsible for memory and cognitive function. In Alzheimer's, less of acetylcholine is present.

Genetics

Genetics plays a large role in this disease. It contributes to the disease in approximately 5–10% of all patients with Alzheimer's. Two types of Alzheimer's include genetic factors; they are called early-onset familial Alzheimer's disease (EOFAD) and late-onset Alzheimer's disease (LOAD).

Early-Onset Familial Alzheimer's Disease

This is when a patient develops Alzheimer's when they are under 65 years old and it is inherited through genes. When specific genes are inherited, Alzheimer's can develop after the age of 65. However, all these cases are quite rare; only 1–5% of patients with Alzheimer's have EOFAD.

Late-Onset Alzheimer's Disease

This is when a patient develops Alzheimer's at an age of over 65 and it is inherited through genes. The difference between the two diseases is that different genes are inherited causing Alzheimer's to be inherited later. Approximately 60–80% of patients with LOAD inherit it through genes.

Dysregulation of Glutamate

Glutamate is a neurotransmitter that normally helps the neurons message each other and follow instructions given by the brain; however, too much glutamate is one of the main factors in Alzheimer's. When glutamate is present in excess, it overuses the neurons, and this can cause damage to the neurons. In dysregulation, the body's immune response is to trigger neuroinflammation, which helps the body. However, too much of it can cause damage to tissues and neurons. Glutamate helps with transmission, which contributes to learning and memory, and too little glutamate can lead to problems with learning and memory, making it harder for patients with Alzheimer's to learn new things and memorise instructions.

Beta-Amyloid Plaques

Beta-amyloid is an example of a protein fragment that forms insoluble clumps outside neurons, such as:

Pyramidal Neurons → Neurons that help with higher cognitive function, such as memory, learning, and decision-making.

Cholinergic Neurons → Neurons that produce a neurotransmitter called acetylcholine, which helps with learning, memory, and attention.

Dopaminergic Neurons → These are less affected, but they help with cognitive function.

Glutamatergic Neurons → These make connections between neurons and produce a neurotransmitter called glutamate.

When these proteins build up, they block the essential needs of the neuron and eventually lead to cell death.

Tau Tangles

Tau is a protein that is normally used to stabilise the internal structure of neurons and ensure that every part of the neuron obtains the nutrients it needs. However abnormal tau proteins become phosphorylated, meaning too much tau is added; this leads to the formation of tau tangles. They can be seen as distorted thin strings inside the neurons. These tau tangles disrupt the supply of nutrients to the cell, eventually leading to cell death.

Neuroinflammation

These are the body's response to the build-up of beta-amyloid plaques and the formation of tau tangles. When the brain senses these, immune cells are activated, and they release chemicals to call more immune cells; after this, inflammatory chemicals are produced that signal more immune cells to the location that requires these cells. However, too much of this inflammatory response would damage tissues as well as neurons and cells.

Oxidative Stress

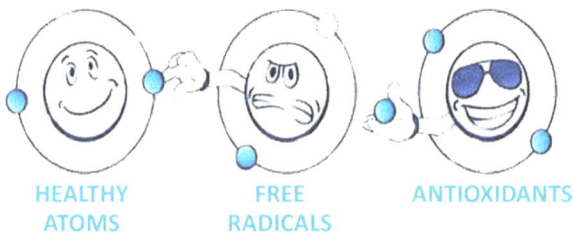

HEALTHY ATOMS   FREE RADICALS   ANTIOXIDANTS

This term describes an imbalance between free radicals and antioxidants. Free radicals have unpaired electrons, and when looking for electrons to fill in the one that is missing, they take them from tissues and cells, which damages them. Antioxidants help keep free radicals from stealing electrons from tissues and cells by giving them electrons while staying stable themselves. When there is an imbalance, free radicals can exceed the number of antioxidants, meaning that they steal electrons from important neurons and cells, which can lead to cell death. This also contributes to the progression of Alzheimer's. The formation of beta-amyloid plaques and tau tangles increases the number of free radicals, causing an imbalance.

Symptoms

Alzheimer's has many symptoms; some are more serious than others, but the end product is always the same.

Memory Loss

Memory loss is one of the most common symptoms of Alzheimer's and is mainly caused because of the build-up of beta-amyloid plaques on neurons, such as the pyramidal neurons and cholinergic neurons mentioned earlier, which contribute to helping people remember important things, including dates and events (for example, a loved one's birthday).

Cognitive Decline

Cognitive decline is a process in which problem-solving skills decrease, and patients cannot solve basic problems. This is because of damage to certain brain cells such as [pyramidal neurons, which help with thinking with common sense. These neurons experience a lack of nutrients due to tau tangles, and other essential needs are blocked by beta-amyloid plaques; this means that the cells are weaker and less able to solve problems that require common sense. This is a common symptom of neurons not functioning properly.

Disorientation

Disorientation is when everything seems foggy and unclear; this is when the most famous symptom of Alzheimer's comes into play, not being able to recognise the familiar faces of loved ones. This is often due to neurotransmitter imbalances—in this case, the dysfunctional release of glutamate. Patients always feel unsafe and unsure of their surroundings, the current time, and where they are.

Difficulty with Daily Tasks

This is when patients find everyday tasks, such as taking a bath, getting dressed, and eating, to be huge challenges. For example, consider someone playing football for the first time in a very long time who is playing in a match in which everyone else knows how to play the game very well. At first, they will find the game hard, with many gaps in the rules and an inability to recall what to do in the game. This is the daily life of an Alzheimer's patient—constantly forgetting essential things in their daily activities. This is because of the dysregulation of the release of neurotransmitters, neurons' inability to react quickly to problems, and the gradual death of neurons that help access essential data due to tau tangles and beta-amyloid plaques.

Changes in Personality

Patients with Alzheimer's are typically depressed, and they feel left out and unsafe most of the time. Imagine a random person coming into your house and socialising with you; they call you by your name, state that they are your close relative, and are alone with you. How would you feel?

Terrified. That is how patients with Alzheimer's feel all the time. This leads to a huge change in their personality, as they are unable to trust anyone, and thus they are normally depressed. Most patients are bedridden, as they forget how to take care of themselves. Memories and past experiences form a huge part of what you are and who you trust. Since the lack of cells and faulty neurotransmitters prevent patients from accessing memories and normal routines, they do not enjoy previous experiences or act like themselves anymore.

Other Symptoms

ALZHEIMER'S SYMPTOMS

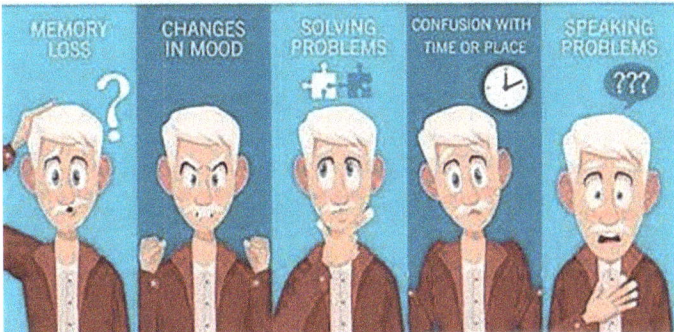

These are some minor symptoms that are branches of the symptoms above:

- Misplacing Items
- Not being comfortable collaborating socially
- Not being very good with problems involving logical thinking and common sense
- Loss of enjoyment of previous hobbies

- Lack of familiarity with things they have done repeatedly
- Often not being able to recall or follow a simple routine
- Difficulty with numbers and problems involving high brain power
- Overall, not very good at subjects like math that involve a lot of thinking and memorising
- Mood swings due to often feeling unsafe and alone

Current Remedies

Many remedies for Alzheimer's are currently available, and they mainly aim to relieve the symptoms and help with daily life despite the difficulties patients face.

Acetylcholinesterase Inhibitors

As mentioned before, acetylcholine is a neurotransmitter that helps communicate with the neurons involved in memory, cognitive function, and learning. Some medicines inhibit these chemicals to help communicate between the neurons temporarily; this is a good temporary fix in the early stages of Alzheimer's and helps manage symptoms; however, later in the disease, far too many factors are present for these inhibitors to handle. They fight the enzymes breaking the acetylcholine, but soon, tau tangles, beta-amyloid plaques, and excessive glutamate are present, along with the inflammation that arises from the body's immune response.

Anti-Amyloid Therapies

These therapies are designed to cling to the beta-amyloid plaques by binding to them, triggering responses to help remove them, preventing their formation temporarily, and slowing the progression a bit. Here are some examples.

Monoclonal Antibodies

These antibodies enter your body, and you can think of them as the physical ones. They bind to the beta-amyloid plaques and remove them by triggering the immune response; these antibodies recognise these protein fragments and then temporarily halt progression. This clears them from the specifically targeted cells.

Beta-Secretase Inhibitors

These inhibitors go straight to where these beta-amyloids are constructed—an enzyme called beta-secretase. These inhibitors are classified as small molecules that block beta-secretase from producing beta-amyloid peptides; when multiple clumps form together around certain neurons, they are called beta-amyloid plaques. Blocking these peptides slows the construction of beta-amyloid plaques straight from the source, which is quite reliable.

Gamma-Secretase Modulators

Gamma-secretase is an enzyme also involved in the production of the protein that makes up the beta-amyloid peptides. These modulators (compounds) help produce fewer toxic forms of beta-amyloid peptides; therefore, the production of beta-amyloid species is decreased, and the other neutral forms then increase.

Anti-Amyloid Vaccine

When injected, these vaccines produce harmless fake molecules that then take the form of beta-amyloid peptides and initiate the human body's immune response of producing antibodies. These fake protein fragments cling to the harmful ones and trigger the antibodies to destroy them both and clear the beta-amyloids around the neurons.

My Favourite Anti-Amyloid Therapies

My favourite anti-amyloid therapy is the beta-secretase inhibitors because they tackle the location where the main production occurs and thus seem to be the most effective. Therefore, they are one of the aspects that I include in my final theory at the end of this explanation of Alzheimer's.

Handling Glutamate Levels

Glutamate is a neurotransmitter; because of its dysregulation, when released, it leads to the build-up of beta-amyloid plaques and tau tangles in the neurons. Here are a few of the current remedies to tackle this problem.

Memantine

Memantine works like a traffic modulator; it helps keep control of the amount of glutamate in the brain. A steady amount is needed because without it, the body would not be able to send messages between neurons. However, because there may be too many aspects to tackle and since it only targets glutamate dysregulation, it might not be as effective. This medicine is normally prescribed in the latter stages of the disease when symptoms are much harder to manage. Memantine helps manage those symptoms, but because Alzheimer's is such a progressive disease, even though it helps with cognitive function temporarily, it could never tackle Alzheimer's alone.

Riluzole

Riluzole is another modulator like memantine; however, instead of controlling the amount of glutamate, it decreases it. Therefore, this is normally prescribed if a greater amount of glutamate is detected in the body, in which case this would be helpful. This medicine has also been investigated for its neuroprotective effects, which help fight against inflammation and other factors that may eventually lead to cell death. Riluzole has been used to enhance GABAergic transmission. GABA stands for gamma-aminobutyric acid; it is a neurotransmitter that contributes to relaxation and helps manage the symptoms of excessive glutamate.

Ketamine

Ketamine is like a bodyguard of a certain type of receptor that acts like a door controlling what enters and exits; sometimes it lets unnecessary information through, which challenges learning and memory. The chemical ketamine makes the receptors sharper so that they only allow the needed information through, enhancing a patient's memory and ability to learn. This helps manage symptoms and enables patients with Alzheimer's to live as well as possible.

Lamotrigine

This chemical is used primarily in diseases such as epilepsy and bipolar disorder, but it has been investigated for its potential in helping with Alzheimer's. This is because it helps with the connections between different neurons. In Alzheimer's, it could potentially help with toxicity, which is when too much glutamate is released from its receptors. Lamotrigine helps fix 'electrical' connections indirectly; it blocks certain channels of neurons to reduce the release of glutamate.

D-Cycloserine

This is a chemical normally used in tuberculosis, but it has been investigated for its possible use and potential in Alzheimer's because it helps keep a receptor that releases glutamate under control so that there is no dysregulation of glutamate releasing and closing all the problems, such as tau tangles and the build-up of beta-amyloid plaques.

The Best Remedy (In My Opinion)

Out of all these chemicals, the ones I have chosen are memantine and riluzole; this is because they are the safest and help with controlling the symptoms of Alzheimer's the most. Memantine helps control glutamate release, and riluzole helps fight against inflammation with its neuroprotective effects and the release of GABA to help the patient relax. In addition, acetylcholinesterase Inhibitors play a crucial role in increasing this neurotransmitter to help manage the symptoms of the disease. I would combine this with my favourite anti-amyloid therapy, beta-secretase inhibitors, to provide a huge relief and effective remedy for Alzheimer's:

Riluzole + acetylcholinesterase inhibitors + memantine + beta-secretase Inhibitors → Handles symptoms well

Huntington's Disease

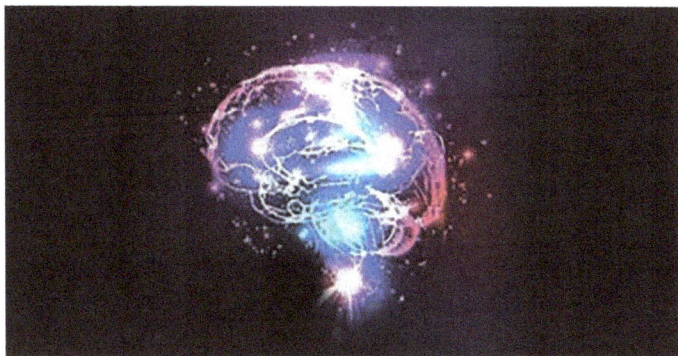

History of Huntingtons

Huntingtons like Parkinson's also dates back quite early into tht 17th century were doctors wrote reports on chorea like movements one of the most famous was the English physician Charles Oscar Water in the mid 1800s, he described this disease in New English families.

In Long Island, New York a man called Charles Gorman also saw a similar pattern in a large family, he noticed that the disease ran through the generations.

In 1872 George Huntington did research on the disease and wrote an essay titled 'On Chorea', this essay talked about how Huntingtons was commonly inherited and it's progressive properties as well as it normally occurring in mid ages like 40-50.

In the 1900's a lot of research was done on Huntington's and many advancements were made, in the 20s and 30s the pattern that parents with Huntingtons gave their children a 50% chance of inheriting it as well.

Later in 1970 the advancement in molecular biology made it easier to locate the chromosome that the mutant gene was in.

In 1993 the major breakthrough of Huntington's was made, linking to the work in 1970 the discovery of the extra CAG repeat in the mutant Huntingtin gene which produces a mutant huntingtin when read by the mRNA which is the root cause of all the problems.

Although there is no cure at the moment, gene editing tools like CRISPR Cas-9 is being used in order to replace the gene. I will give you a deeper insight into the disease and the current treatments to help cope with symptoms and remove the mutant gene.

What is Huntington's Disease and what Causes It?

Huntington's disease is a neurodegenerative disease that originates from a problem in the genes. It is caused when the protein Huntingtin, which helps with neuronal signals and normal cell function, is replaced with a mutant gene that causes abruption in the body, damages cell function neuronal signals, and more, immensely. Huntington's can affect people of various ages, but it more commonly affects earlier age groups (around 20–40 years old), It occurs only because of the mutant huntingtin; research has shown that people who have Huntington's and reproduce have a 50% chance of having children with Huntington's. Huntington's is a neurodegenerative disease involving many factors, such as mitochondria dysfunction, the build-up of insoluble aggregates, and the disruption of nutrients from entering the cells. One of the main reasons it is neurodegenerative is that, as genes are in the nucleus of all cells, the infected mutant gene is present in each cell, causing these problems in each cell.

What is Huntingtin?

As mentioned above, Huntingtin is a protein that normally helps with the function of healthy neurons and helps mitochondria provide energy to the cell and keep it alive.

The protein also helps ensure that the transport of cargo and organelles through the microtubules (like roads in the cell) runs smoothly. Huntingtin plays a key role in synapses, where the neurotransmitters are released and the neurons communicate with each other; an insufficient number of these proteins could cause severe problems with memory and learning.

Structure of the Mutant Huntingtin Gene

The mutant huntingtin gene is what accumulates into large groups and causes neuronal dysfunction and cell death. This is the definition of Huntington's. To form an adequate theory to combat Huntington's disease, this disease must be thoroughly understood. This gene is made up of four structures—the polyglutamine tract, the N terminal region, the C terminal region, and HEAT repeats. Below, I delve into each component in detail.

Polyglutamine Tract (PolyQ tract)

This tract is the stem of all the problems in Huntington's disease. The tract holds something called a CAG (cytosine–adenine–guanine, the three bases of nucleotides), and this sequence repeats itself in the DNA sequence. CAG normally repeats around 10–35 times in a healthy person, but in patients with Huntington's, it repeats over 36 times, the more the CAG repeats, the earlier a patient is more prone to the disease, as it shows that the mutant huntingtin is present. This tract with the mutant huntingtin is longer than usual. Huntington's is known to be neurodegenerative like Alzheimer's and Parkinson's because when the cells split, the tract expands and contracts, and therefore, it is replicated because of the division of cells.

N Terminal Region

This is what contains the PolyQ tract, and it is involved in various protein interactions and cellular processes. When the CAG sequence is extended, the starting point for these interactions is altered, meaning the signal at the start of the N terminal (the start of the whole gene because the N terminal is the start of the whole gene) could mislead the cells, and the pathways could be disrupted, leading to mayhem in the cells. The extended N terminal region also may not bind to the right molecules/proteins; this could cause a variety of problems, such as proteins being led to the wrong place as well as the folding and clumping of the protein, which can disrupt the cellular function and form aggregates. These clumps are often toxic to the cell and lead to their dysfunction and eventually death. The proteins that are needed for the cells' survival are not being able to perform their function.

HEAT Repeats

The HEAT repeats are in the middle of the mutant huntingtin, and this normally allows for correctly ordered proteins. However, in the mutant, this is disrupted; the repeats interact like Lego building blocks joined together with different proteins, and when this fails, the structure changes, causing the protein to misfold and not interact properly with other proteins. These repeats enhance the production of the toxic aggregates by the proteins and the clumping of the mutant huntingtin. In a proper huntingtin protein, these HEAT repeats play a large role in the transport of nutrients into the cells, but with the mutant protein, these nutrient transports are disrupted.

C Terminal Region

The C Terminal is at the back of the gene on the opposite end of the N terminal region; it basically performs the same functions as the N terminal region but at the opposite end of the gene strand.

Symptoms

Some of the early symptoms are difficulty concentrating, memory lapses, depression, stumbling and clumsiness, and mood swings. A few of the later symptoms are involuntary jerking, difficulty speaking clearly, trouble swallowing, increasingly slow movements, changes in personality, problems with breathing, and difficulty moving around.

Early Symptoms

Difficulty Concentrating

Difficulty concentrating is one of the early symptoms because it is due to the degeneration of neurons in places such as the basal ganglia and hippocampus. The basal ganglia is a set of nuclei in the brain that is in charge of coordinating and executing movement, and they are also involved in reward processing, which helps with managing emotions. The hippocampus is responsible for memories and managing short- and long-term memories. In my opinion, the cortex plays a vital role in this symptom because it is in control of attentiveness and language. Language comes into play as a later symptom. The degeneration of neurons in these important aspects of the brain leads to memory lapses, which shows that the disease progression might be a bit deeper. Memory lapses are a common symptom in Alzheimer's, but they are also common in mild Huntington's, as this disease shows steady degeneration in the hippocampus. These lapses restrict patients from remembering important dates and events, such as birthdays, along with their routines.

Depression

As mentioned earlier, the basal ganglia is in charge of reward processing and works alongside neurotransmitters, such as dopamine and glutamate. Dopamine is normally classified as the reward hormone, and the dysregulation of dopamine could cause this depression. Like the previous symptom, depression is normally caused by the degeneration of neurons in a certain area, such as the basal ganglia, and the dysregulation of glutamate and dopamine release, which affects mood regulation.

Stumbling and Clumsiness

This symptom is also due to the degeneration of neurons in the basal ganglia and cortex. Stumbling and clumsiness could be considered the basis of a much more severe symptom called chorea, which I will expand on later. Cortical regions in the brain, such as the motor cortex, are responsible for planning and initiating movements. The degeneration of cortical neurons in the brain makes the patient more prone to falling, slipping, and tripping. When you were a toddler, your parents may have had you put coins in a tin box with a slit or tell you to put a thread into a needle; these are activities that increase your fine motor skills. In Huntington's, these skills are affected, which results in the patient being more clumsy. Huntington's also leads to the progressive degeneration of motor and sensory pathways, which could send delayed signals about the terrain and where the patient is placing his or her foot next.

Late Symptoms

Chorea

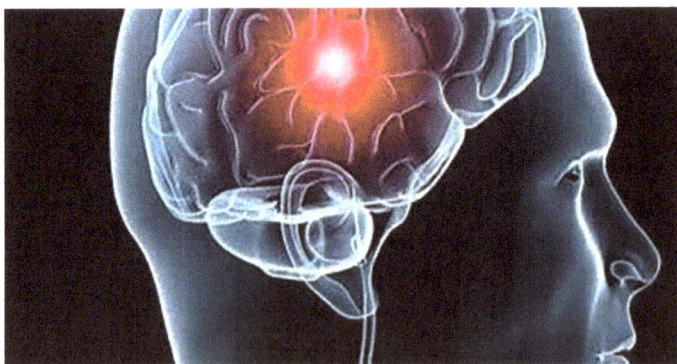

Chorea is the term for random uncontrollable movements that affect many parts of the body, particularly the limbs; this is noted as a common symptom in Parkinson's but is displayed in severe Huntington's as well. As mentioned before, Huntington's affects the basal ganglia and degenerates it, and the basal ganglia controls the body and movement. Chorea is involved when there is more degeneration in that part of the body. Chorea is involved in the degeneration of certain neurons; these neurons work together in a circuit to perform certain movements and actions. However, the degeneration of these neurons disrupts the neuron circuits and thus disrupts these movements, causing fluctuations and impaired movement.

Difficulty Speaking Clearly

This symptom consists of changes in the voice, less articulation when speaking, and not speaking very loudly. Speaking clearly is part of the job of the basal ganglia, and as it degenerates, the muscles involved in speaking and changing the voice tone become more rigid. This results in slurred speech and quiet voices, words often coming out unclear, and an inability to speak with different tones and pitches. Memory also plays a part in speaking clearly; as huntingtin degenerates neurons responsible for long- and short-term memory, the retrieval of words becomes difficult. A muscle called the laryngeal muscle is affected, which helps with the quality of the voice; alongside this, vocal cord dysfunction due to muscle rigidity results in a strained voice.

Swallowing Problems

The basal ganglia is involved in swallowing, and the degeneration of neurons in that area disrupts the neuronal circuits, resulting in swallowing problems. There is also reduced control of bolus (food and drink) in the mouth, as the cheek and mouth muscles do not act as swiftly, causing trouble with coordinating the food and an inability to swallow as effectively as a normal person.

Personality Changes

All of these symptoms have a mental impact on the patient, making them not feel included or like themselves anymore;

the mutant huntingtin also affects the dysregulation of neurotransmitters, such as dopamine and glutamate, which affects mood and personality. As mentioned earlier, depression is one of the early symptoms, and mood swings and personality changes follow, as emotions are not processed as effectively. Because of long- and short-term memory problems, people might not be able to recognise others, and this would cause problems with socialising. They are more prone to mood swings because of the dysregulation of neurotransmitters, and the degeneration of many neurons involved in decision-making could lead to quick decisions that are not given much thought.

Current Cures and Remedies

A few remedies have been used to combat the merciless symptoms that make the lives of people with Huntington's so difficult.

Physiotherapy

The book *The Man Who Mistook His Wife for a Hat* highlights the uses of physiotherapy in diseases. Physiotherapy is all about trying to trick your brain into believing that you are already cured and countering symptoms of diseases through certain exercises. This is a common therapy in many neurodegenerative diseases such as Huntington's, but it is used across the entire field, which includes Parkinson's and Alzheimer's. This can be used to counter symptoms such as chorea by stretching the hands and legs; it can also be used to help with coordination, which is a major problem in the disease. Functional exercises help with simple daily exercises, such as walking up the stairs and going for walks; under the supervision of a professional, these exercises can help give the patient more independence. Manual therapy (another subset) is used to help alleviate pain through a series of massages and joint exercises; these help the connective tissues move better, helping the patient move more easily.

Tetrabenazine

This medicine is used to help control the effects of chorea in Huntington's, but it is quite dangerous and can be too effective, meaning that it may even lead to serious symptoms of Parkinson's. Parkinson's is relevant here because this medicine stops VMAT2, which is a type of packaging chemical, from putting too much dopamine into vesicles (like little bags) to be transported around the body. Too much dopamine causes these involuntary movements, but not enough dopamine leads to symptoms of Parkinson's. This medicine must be prescribed by a doctor, as it could lead to depression and suicidal thoughts if used too much because dopamine is key for happiness.

Antipsychotic Medications

Under this type of medication are two other medications that I thought would be useful in Huntington's: haloperidol and risperidone. These medications also target the production of too much dopamine to help balance the dopamine levels in the brain.

Haloperidol and Risperidone: Similarities and Differences

Haloperidol works by attaching to the D-2 receptors, which produce dopamine. These receptors are what dopamine binds to, and they then become effective and serve their purpose. When haloperidol binds these receptors, it blocks the dopamine from clinging to the receptors, as there is already too much of it in the body, resulting in hallucinations (e.g., seeing things that no one else sees and hearing things that no one else hears). Risperidone, on the other hand, binds to D-2 receptors and serotonin receptors. Serotonin is involved in controlling mood and emotions; blocking these receptors limits serotonin, meaning that patients can cope better with mood swings in Huntington's. I think risperidone is more effective, as it is used in a variety of disorders, such as schizophrenia and autism.

Stem Cells

You may have heard of these types of cells before as they are very popular and I simply couldn't miss writing about this in a book about neurodegenerative diseases.

Stem cells are unspecialized and have no sort of specific function, however they are classified as pluripotent meaning Stem Cells can change into any type of cell in your body whether if its a fat cell, a muscle cell or even a neuron. These types of cells have been explored before especially in the context of many diseases such as the ones we discussed so far, one of the most famous applications of this is in the disease leukaemia. This is a disease effecting the bone marrow were stem cells to become blood cells are produced, the cells grow uncontrollably into cancer cells overcrowding the stem cells and causing terrible damage to the blood cells produced. Patients that got an injection of stem cells that formed into healthy blood cells were able to restore the amount of blood cells needed and overall restore the health of the patient.

There are many ethical problems to this as there has been no new technology to create artificial stem cells, so like a heart transplant there would be a stem cell transplant from another persons body, the stem cells would be taken from the bone marrow of another patient and transferred to the patient that needs it. This could increase the risk of an donor getting a disease like leukaemia and would be defenceless against it.

Stem cells can be found in many parts of your body such as the:

- Lining of intestine
- Stem cells in blood marrow
- Stem cells in the umbilical cord which can be stored from birth for future use
- Stem cells on the skin used for regeneration of skin
- Stem cells in the liver which can be regenerated when liver is infected with some diseases
- Stem cells in muscle to help increase their size and better function
- Stem cells in areas of brain such as the hippocampus to help complete neural circuits

There are two types of stem cells the first is Somatic stem cells which are found in the parts of the body like bone marrow and hippocampus which are multipotent meaning they can be transformed into many types of cells but not as many as the Embryonic stem cells that are found in the blastocyst stage of a developing embryo.

The excitement is that Somatic stem cells might be able to transform into more cells than we think which could help replace in the Parkinson's context the dopamine producing neurons and in the Alzheimer's context the glutamatergic neurons and much more. This holds a lot of promise and is an important research medicine that scientists are currently deeply exploring.

Final Conclusion

Thank you for reading my book and embarking on this journey with me through the interesting world of neurodegenerative diseases. I hope you have enjoyed this book and gained more insights into the world of the brain.

Sources

Parkinson's Disease | National Institute of Neurological Disorders and Stroke (nih.gov)

Parkinson's disease - NHS (www.nhs.uk)

Pramipexole - Wikipedia

Ropinirole: treats the symptoms of Parkinson's disease - NHS (www.nhs.uk)

Rotigotine - Wikipedia

Apomorphine | Parkinson's UK (parkinsons.org.uk)

Omega-3 Fatty Acids & the Important Role They Play (clevelandclinic.org)

Health Benefits of Resveratrol — And Should You Take It? (clevelandclinic.org)

What is curcumin | Holland & Barrett (hollandandbarrett. com)

Pentoxifylline Neuroprotective Effects Are Possibly Related to Its Anti-Inflammatory and TNF-Alpha Inhibitory Properties, in the 6-OHDA Model of Parkinson's Disease (hindawi.com) (1)

Liposomal Formulations in Clinical Use: An Updated Review - PMC (nih.gov)

Alzheimer's Association

Alzheimer's disease - NHS (www.nhs.uk)

Acetylcholinesterase inhibitors | Prescribing information | Dementia | CKS | NICE

Production of monoclonal antibodies - Higher Tier - Monoclonal antibodies - Higher - AQA - GCSE Biology (Single Science) Revision - AQA - BBC Bitesize

BACE1 (β-secretase) inhibitors for the treatment of Alzheimer's disease - PubMed (nih.gov)

CAS 937812-80-1 gamma-Secretase modulators - BOC Sciences

Is the 100-year old TB vaccine a new weapon against Alzheimer's? | Alzheimer's | The Guardian

About memantine - NHS (www.nhs.uk)

Riluzole | Drugs | BNF | NICE

Ketamine | Effects of Ketamine | FRANK (talktofrank.com)

Lamotrigine: medicine to treat epilepsy and bipolar disorder - NHS (www.nhs.uk)

D-Cycloserine in Neuropsychiatric Diseases: A Systematic Review - PMC (nih.gov)

Methylene Blue solution alkaline according to Loeffler according to Loeffler 61-73-4 (sigmaaldrich.com)

ANAVEX2-73 for Treatment of Early Alzheimer's Disease - Full Text View - ClinicalTrials.gov

Microbubbles and ultrasound: from diagnosis to therapy | European Heart Journal - Cardiovascular Imaging | Oxford Academic (oup.com)

The Myth of Equipoise in Phase 1 Clinical Trials - PMC (nih.gov)

Huntington's disease - NHS (www.nhs.uk)

N-Terminal Regions of Prion Protein: Functions and Roles in Prion Diseases - PMC (nih.gov)

Polyglutamine (polyQ) disorders - PMC (nih.gov)

HEAT Repeats Associated with Condensins, Cohesins, and Other Complexes Involved in Chromosome-Related Functions - PMC (nih.gov)

Physiotherapy - NHS (www.nhs.uk)

Tetrabenazine | Drugs | BNF | NICE

Risperidone | Drugs | BNF | NICE

7.21A: Chemotaxis - Biology LibreTexts

DNA Ligase- Definition, Structure, Types, Functions (microbenotes.com)

National Center for Biotechnology Information (NCBI): Liver Regeneration

Harvard Stem Cell Institute: Liver

National Institute of Neurological Disorders and Stroke (NINDS): Neural Stem Cells

NIH National Institute on Aging: Neurogenesis

National Center for Biotechnology Information (NCBI): Satellite Cells

University of Michigan Medicine: Satellite Cells

About the Author

My name is Joshua Dominique, and I am 11 years old. I have been interested in the field of neurology for a few years and now I have written a book on the three main neurodegenerative diseases. This book is only to spark interest in many others about neurology and spread the message that these diseases are out there, and we need more people to help find the cures. I am taking the first step in proclaiming this to the outside world and inviting people to enter the interesting realm of neurology. This book covers the basics of each disease and the factors that contribute to another factor that eventually can cause difficulty living or death to the patient. I hope this book inspires you to explore neurology and embark on this journey with me.

www.ingramcontent.com/pod-product-compliance
Lightning Source LLC
Chambersburg PA
CBHW042119190326
41519CB00030B/7549